GW01072077

Clinical Manual on
VAGINAL CANDIDOSIS
1994

Clinician's Manual on
VAGINAL CANDIDOSIS
1994

GR Kinghorn

Department of Genitourinary Medicine
Royal Hallamshire Hospital
Sheffield UK

SCIENCE PRESS

© Copyright 1994 by Science Press Limited, 34–42 Cleveland Street, London, W1P 5FB, UK

British Library Cataloguing in Publication Data
A catalogue record for this book is available from the British Library.

ISBN 1-85873-010-4

This copy of the *Clinician's Manual on Vaginal Candosis* is given as a service to medicine by Pfizer. Sponsorship of this copy does not imply the sponsor's agreement or otherwise with the views expressed herein.

Although every effort has been made to ensure that drug doses and other information are presented accurately in this publication, the ultimate responsibility rests with the prescribing physician. Neither the publishers nor the authors can be held responsible for errors or for any consequences arising from the use of the information contained therein. Any product mentioned in this publication should be used in accordance with the prescribing information prepared by the manufacturers. No claims or endorsements are made for any drug or compound.

Project editors: Hilary Michie and Alison Taylor
Illustrator: Paul Bernson
Typesetters: Paul Angliss and Tanya Mukerjee
Production: Rebecca Spencer
Printed in Hong Kong by Paramount Printing Company Ltd.

Contents

Contents

5 Drug treatment of VVC

Acknowledgements

Page 32
Adapted by permission from *Fluconazole and its role in vaginal candidosis* (Richardson RG, ed.). Royal Society of Medicine Services, London, 1989

Page 33
Adapted by permission from International Multicentre Trial. *Br J Obstet Gynaecol* 96: 22, 1989

Page 34
Adapted by permission from Kutzer E, Oitter R, Leudolter S, Brammer KW: *Eur J Gynaecol Reprod Biol* 29: 305, 1988

INTRODUCTION

Within the wide spectrum of human fungal diseases, vaginal candidosis may be viewed by some clinicians as being trivial in comparison with the serious systemic mycoses which occur in severely immunocompromised patients. Yet it is a common gynaecological condition which affects many women at some time in their lives and is treated by both hospital specialists and general practitioners alike.

Much remains to be understood about the host factors which allow yeasts, which are normally part of the commensal flora in many areas of the body, to become invasive and initiate inflammatory disease. Despite the availability of a number of effective (and now safe) topical and orally active drugs, the management of this disorder in some women who suffer from chronic and recurring symptoms often proves extremely challenging to clinicians.

I hope that this handbook will provide doctors with an insight into the complexity of vaginal candidosis and prove to be a useful and practical management guide to the benefit of their patients.

GR Kinghorn
1994

1 WHAT IS VAGINAL CANDIDOSIS?

1.1 Definition

Vaginal candidosis, also known as vulvovaginal candidosis (VVC), is an inflammatory disease of the vulva and vagina caused by yeast infection. The disease is known in Europe as candidal vaginitis and, in the USA and Canada, as vulvovaginal candidiasis. Moniliasis is the older and now defunct name. In many countries, the condition is also known as 'thrush'.

1.2 Prevalence and impact

VVC is very common worldwide. It has been estimated that 75% of adult women from all socioeconomic strata will suffer from the condition at some time in their life. It is rare in premenarchal and postmenopausal women. In most individuals, the disorder is little more than a temporary annoyance and inconvenience. In a minority, however, the disease is chronic and/or recurrent (four times per year or more) and may have serious consequences for the patient's quality of life. The constant itch, burning and discharge may provoke major psychological and psychosocial disturbances. Sexual dysfunction often accompanies these symptoms and discord within a relationship may ensue.

Incidence

Asymptomatic genital colonization and symptomatic infection of the vagina are more common in patients attending sexually transmitted disease (STD) clinics than in the general population. The annual increase in new cases of VVC at clinics in England between 1976 and 1990 was 70%.

1.3 Organism distribution

Candida albicans and related species are yeasts — fungi that possess a predominantly unicellular mode of development. There are over 150 species within this genus which occur in most terrestrial and aquatic environments. Those associated with human disease represent only a minority subset of a large heterogeneous group and occur primarily in man and warm blooded animals usually as part of the commensal flora of their gastrointestinal (GI) tracts. *C. albicans* has a wider range of animal hosts than other pathogenic species. It can also be isolated from inanimate objects subject to human and animal contamination and is used as an indicator of pollution in sea-water. It survives poorly on dry surfaces but is more resistant in moist conditions. *C. albicans* can survive on toothbrushes, underwear, in hand-cream and other oil–water based cosmetics.

Vulvovaginal candidosis

C. albicans and other yeasts can cause a variety of human diseases, including penile candidosis, cystitis, napkin rash and systemic infection.

Clinical spectrum of diseases associated with *Candida* species	
Disease	**Sources/transmission**
Vulvovaginal candidosis	Vagina
Penile candidosis	
Neonatal oral candidosis	
Infected burns	Oral-cutaneous
Panonychia	
Candida cystitis	Faecal spread
Napkin rash	
Systemic candidosis	Gastrointestinal tract

1.4 Causative species

C. albicans has been isolated from more than 80% of specimens obtained from women with VVC. Approximately 20% of sexually active women carry the identical *Candida* strain in their GI tract and vagina.

The incidence of VVC in STD clinics in the UK between 1976 and 1992 is shown in the figure opposite. Many more cases are

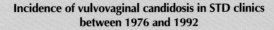

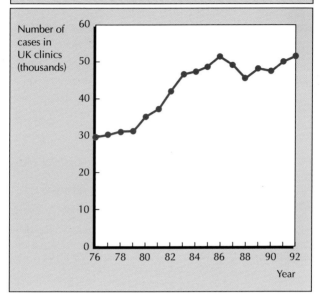

Incidence of vulvovaginal candidosis in STD clinics between 1976 and 1992

Number of cases in UK clinics (thousands)

Year

treated by general practitioners but no comparable statistics are available from this source. The total number of prescriptions issued for treatment of VVC in 1992 was in excess of 3 million.

C. glabrata (formerly known as *Torulopsis glabrata*), which is more resistant to treatment, is responsible for about 5% of cases. Because there is a tendency for *C. glabrata* to be selected out by some of the azole drugs, particularly ketoconazole, an increase in the number of positive isolates is to be expected. *C. tropicalis* and *C. parapsilosis* are usually found in association with systemic infections; rarer isolates include *C. kefyr*, *C. krusei* and *Saccharomyces cerevisiae* (Baker's yeast).

1.5 Carriage rates for *C. albicans*
Candida species can be found in many areas of the body within healthy individuals. Differences in the selection of individuals, sampling and culture techniques influence the reported carriage rates.

Yeast concentrations are usually lower in healthy carriers than in women with disease. The carriage rates for the GI tract (mouth, stomach, small intestine, rectum) and vagina are greater than 50% and 10–20%, respectively. Penile carriage within the general population is uncommon but up to 33% of partners of infected women are also affected.

In most individuals the biotype of the pathogen will be the same as that of a commensal organism found at an alternative body site.

2 AETIOLOGY AND PATHOGENESIS

2.1 Morphology of yeasts

All pathogenic yeasts multiply primarily by the production of buds from a small selected site on their cell surface (blastospores). The sizes and shapes of the spores are sometimes characteristic of a species.

Some yeasts also form chains of elongated, unseparated blastospores or pseudohyphae. *C. albicans* can also form true hyphae (microscopic tubes that contain multiple fungal cell units divided by septa) in addition to large refractory chlamydospores (large refractive thick walled cells formed in response to nutrient depletion).

Blastospores predominate in secretions in which the organism is considered to be commensal. In infected human tissues, a mixture of budding yeasts, pseudohyphae and true hyphae are seen. Conditions which favour the formation of the filamentous forms of *Candida* include

- high CO_2 concentrations

- partial anaerobiasis

- temperature $< 35^{o}C$

- pH $> 6.5–7.0$

- growth in liquid media

Structure and composition of *Candida* species

Electron microscopy of pathogenic *Candida* species reveals a multilayered cell wall. The cell wall serves two unique functions: it maintains the cell shape and it is the site of contact between the fungus and its environment. Differences in the ability of *C. albicans* strains to alter their shape and to adhere to host surfaces may be virulence attributes.

The yeast is made up of 20–40% proteins, 30–50% polysaccharides, and varying proportions of lipids. The amount of lipid and its composition varies according to the strain, culture age, and environmental conditions. Phospholipids and sterols are dominant, with ergosterol being the predominant sterol.

6

2.2 Growth and nutrition of pathogenic *Candida* species

Most *Candida* species grow well in aerobic cultures on nutrient media, in broad pH and temperature ranges. All pathogenic species have their optimal growth temperature nearer 37°C than do non-pathogenic species. They will also grow under elevated concentrations of CO_2 in air. Growth rates vary according to the strain and the growth conditions used. Under optimal conditions, the doubling time is about one hour.

The pathogenic *Candida* species usually die within a few minutes if they are exposed to temperatures above 50°C. They are also rapidly killed by ultraviolet light.

2.3 Organism factors in pathogenesis

Adhesion

Adherence to epithelial cells is a necessary first step for invasive disease. The ability of a *Candida* species to adhere to epithelial cells is indicative of the relative pathogenicity of that strain. *C. albicans* has the highest rate of adherence of all the yeasts.

Dimorphism

The hyphal form plays an important role in the initial processes of tissue invasion because it is more effective than the yeast cell in adhering to the vaginal epithelium. Both morphological forms have the ability to initiate and sustain pathological responses in mammalian hosts, but it is likely that one particular form is better adapted to survive in specific ecological microniches *in vivo*. The facility for flexible interconversion between these morphological forms confers a heightened degree of pathogenicity.

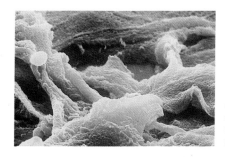

Candida invading exfoliated vaginal epithelial cells (scanning electron microscope).

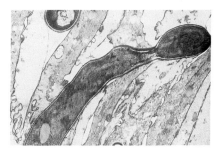

Candida invading vaginal epithelial cells (transmission electron microscope).

Phenotypic switching

C. albicans frequently gives rise to colonial variants in response to ultraviolet light exposure in sublethal doses and adverse growth environments. Smooth, rough, ring, star, wrinkle, fuzzy and stippled colony types are described, which have different proportions of blastospore and filamentous forms and have altered physiological properties. High frequency switching of colony types of *Candida* isolates grown at 24°C has been found more often among strains associated with clinical disease than from strains considered to be commensals. It has been suggested that rapid phenotypic switching may account for the ability of *C. albicans* to invade a large range of environmentally different body sites. It may also be related to changes in antifungal susceptibility.

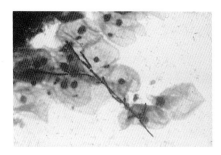

Gram stain of vaginal secretion in acute VVC showing hyphae and blastospores.

Other factors

The production of glycoproteins and other high- and low-molecular-weight toxins by *C. albicans* has been described. The species also produce a broad spectrum of exoenzymes, especially acid proteases and phospholipases, which are able to initiate tissue invasion. Although there are likely to be differences between strains in their relative abilities to produce toxins and exoenzymes, current understanding of their roles as virulence factors remains imprecise.

2.4 Host factors in pathogenesis

Many authorities consider that some change, local or systemic, in patient susceptibility is necessary before *Candida* can act as an opportunistic pathogen and cause inflammatory disease.

Local conditions

In patients whose vagina is colonized by *C. albicans*, inflammatory disease often follows either localized minor trauma or change in the resident bacterial flora (bacteria frustrate yeast growth by interfering with nutrition and by producing growth inhibiting factors).

Humoral immunity to *Candida*

The yeast burden is not necessarily related to the occurrence of symptoms. Hypersensitivity to *Candida* antigens may be important for symptom production in men and women with low yeast loads. Elevated serum and vaginal *Candida*-specific IgE antibody levels have been described in some women with recurrent VVC.

Mucosal antibody secretion involves a complex system in which IgA predominates. High vaginal levels of secretory IgA reduce the adherence of *Candida* to epithelial cells and so lessen the attack rate of associated vaginitis. Some women with recurrent disease have low secretory IgA levels.

Deficiencies in humoral immunity have little significance in the pathogenesis of genital candidosis.

Cellular immunity to *Candida*

In conditions associated with impaired T-lymphocyte cell function, such as haematological malignancy or HIV infection, the incidence and severity of *Candida* mucocutaneous disease is increased.

The glycoprotein of *Candida* has been shown in animal models to suppress normal cellular immune responses.

In most affected women, delayed hypersensitivity responses to multiple antigens, including *Candida,* are normal. In some women with chronic vaginitis, impaired cellular immune responses and *Candida*-specific suppressor lymphocytes, which block the cellular immune response to *Candida* antigens, have been found. An abnormal macrophage interaction with *Candida* antigens resulting in an excess of prostaglandin E_2, which then inhibits the lymphocyte proliferative response, has also been demonstrated. This defect can be overcome *in vitro* by prostaglandin inhibitors, such as ibuprofen. These drugs may have a role as possible adjuncts to conventional antifungal therapy in patients with recurrent candidosis.

3 PREDISPOSING FACTORS

Many systemic and local conditions have been recognized as predisposing to VVC. Recent research has suggested that local factors, especially the effect of restrictive clothing, may be less important than previously thought in the pathogenesis of VVC. Nevertheless, they still retain importance in exacerbating the symptoms associated with the condition.

Predisposing factors for Candidal infections	
Systemic	**Local**
Pregnancy	Poor hygiene
Immunosuppression	Close-fitting garments
DiGeorge syndrome	Nylon underwear
Chronic illness	Obesity
Malignancy	Skin sensitizers
HIV infection	Antiseptics
Metabolic conditions	Deodorants
Diabetes mellitus	Trauma
Endocrine disorders (thyroid, parathyroid, adrenal)	Sexual intercourse
	Excoriation
Iron-deficiency anaemia	Vulval dermatoses
Drugs	
Antibiotics	
Steroids	

3.1 Systemic factors

Pregnancy

The rate of vaginal colonization increases during pregnancy in addition to the incidence of inflammatory disease, especially during the last trimester when typical therapy is less effective.

The glycogen content of vaginal cells is increased in response to high circulating hormone levels. This enhances the proliferation, germination and adherence of *C. albicans*. Yeast growth may also be directly stimulated by the high hormone levels. There is also a decrease in cell-mediated immunity during the last trimester, which further predisposes to symptomatic disease.

Immunosuppression

Suppression of T-cell function by drugs, such as corticosteroids and cytotoxic agents, or systemic disease such as acquired immunodeficiency syndrome (AIDS) or haematological malignancy, or in association with cachexia and weight loss, predisposes to both vaginal candidosis and invasive fungal infection.

Metabolic disorders

Glycosuria and increased glucose concentrations in the vaginal secretions enhance the growth of yeasts in diabetic patients. In non-diabetic women, onset of symptoms can occasionally be related to a dietary, carbohydrate indiscretion. There is, however, little evidence that diet plays an important role in the majority of affected women unless they are overweight.

Chronic mucocutaneous candidiasis is associated with endocrine disorders such as hypothyroidism and hypoparathyroidism, and with iron deficiency and other anaemias. Whether these conditions also predispose to vaginal candidosis is disputed.

Antibiotic therapy

Symptomatic vaginal candidosis is frequent following antibiotic therapy. Antibiotics act by reducing, either absolutely or relatively, the normal population of commensal bacteria which normally frustrate yeast growth. The rate of vaginal colonization and extent of inflammatory disease are considerably increased. Rectal colonization also occurs and may subsequently act as a reservoir for vaginal reinfection. This is most likely with broad-spectrum antibiotics such as ampicillin, cephalosporins, tetracyclines and macrolides. Nevertheless, all antibiotics have some propensity to induce vaginal candidosis.

Women with a history of antibiotic-induced vaginal candidosis may be offered prophylactic anti-candidal pessary/ suppository treatment (which can be conveniently used on alternate days) during the course of subsequent antibiotic therapy.

Oral contraceptives

Symptomatic episodes of VVC in non-pregnant women were shown in the late 1960s to be much more common in women who used oral contraceptives. However, these studies were undertaken with the early high-oestrogen-content pills and did not allow for differences between sexual activity in oral contraceptive users and the control groups.

More recent studies suggest that the modern low-oestrogen-content pills may be associated with higher vaginal yeast carriage rates but have little effect upon the incidence of symptomatic disease.

Most clinicians consider that other preventive measures should be exhausted before advocating an alternative method of contraception in oral-contraceptive users.

3.2 Local factors

- The production of warm, moist, macerated skin through wearing tight clothing and underwear (especially if made of synthetic fibres)

- Obesity

- Incorrect toilet habit (which may lead to yeast colonization being transferred from the anorectum to the vagina)

- Low-temperature washing powders (which fail to kill yeasts contaminating underwear)

- Skin sensitization by vaginal sprays and deodorants

- Chemotrauma from chlorinated swimming pools

- Minor physical damage (especially from tampons, which

may destroy the integrity of the epithelium and predispose to infection)

There is an association between inflammatory disease and sexual intercourse in about 15% of patients; minor trauma of the skin or mucosal surfaces is responsible. Many women with recurrent infection complain of dyspareunia even when mycologically free of infection. If they are not adequately prepared for sexual intercourse, the relative vaginal dryness may predispose to mucocutaneous trauma with subsequent reinfection.

These women often benefit from the temporary use of vaginal lubricants in the immediate post-treatment period.

4 CLINICAL ASPECTS

4.1 Symptoms and signs

Symptoms

The cardinal symptom of VVC is itch which is worse at night and exacerbated by warmth. Burning vulval discomfort, external dysuria and superficial dyspareunia are common accompanying complaints. Excessive thick vaginal discharge is not invariably present. The absence of a fishy odour helps to distinguish the condition from bacterial vaginosis.

There may be a history of a predisposing condition, such as recent antibiotic therapy. Many patients with recurrent candidosis experience a premenstrual symptom exacerbation followed by spontaneous amelioration afterwards. Some women are unable to use tampons because of introital soreness. A patient's subjective symptoms alone, however, are of poor predictive value in the diagnosis of VVC.

Signs

The extent and severity of the physical signs are highly variable. Classically, the vulva and vagina are inflamed, hot and sore; inflamed skin often appears smooth and shiny. Perivulval intertrigo and satellite, vesicular or pustular lesions may be present. The signs may be confined to the vulva. Conversely, vulvitis can be minimal and fissures at the introitus and perineum can be the only abnormality.

The gentle insertion of a speculum may disclose mycotic plaques on the cervix and vaginal walls. The discharge usually has a curd-like or cheesy consistency. Some women develop a profuse watery discharge and vulval oedema, a clinical appearance similar to that of trichomoniasis. This is more often seen in adolescent girls.

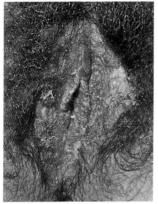

Acute candidal vulvitis.

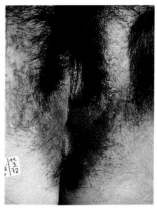

Candidal vulvitis with satellite lesions.

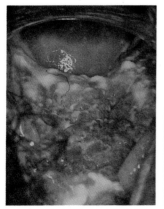

Candidal vaginitis with mycotic plaques.

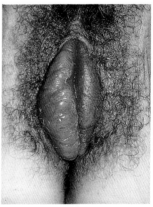

Atypical VVC with oedema.

4.2 Confirmatory tests

A reliable diagnosis cannot be made from the history alone and the physical signs in milder cases are easily misdiagnosed. *C. albicans* frequently coexists with other genital infections.

Office-based tests in vaginal infections			
Test	Vulvovaginal candidosis	Bacterial vaginosis	Trichomoniasis
Vaginal pH	Usually < 4.5	Usually > 5.0	Usually >5.0
KOH 'whiff-test'	Negative	Positive	Variable
Microscopy wet-film	Yeast elements seen	'Clue-cells' seen	Motile tricho-monads seen
Gram smear	Lactobacilli present Gram-positive hyphae and spores	Lactobacilli absent Gram-variable coccobacilli	Lactobacilli often absent Inflammatory cells abound
Culture	Isolation on Sabouraud's medium	Fastidious organisms Not often attempted	Special media desirable

Office-based tests

Testing the vaginal pH, performing a 'whiff-test' (the addition of a drop of 10% potassium hydroxide solution to vaginal secretions on a glass slide releases a fishy amine smell when positive), and microscopic examination of wet film and/or Gram stain preparation of vaginal secretions are very helpful in distinguishing between the causes of vaginal infection.

Filamentous forms are more likely to be seen when *C. albicans* is causing symptomatic invasive disease. The experienced microscopist will make the diagnosis in about 80% of cases with a specificity that approaches 100%.

Candida can also be identified within Papanicolaou-stained cervical cytology smears although the sensitivity is only 30%.

Laboratory isolation methods

Isolation of a yeast in culture is the definitive and sensitive proof of the presence of a yeast in a clinical specimen.

Although it is more sensitive than microscopy, it does not differentiate between commensal and pathogenic flora. Cotton-tipped swabs are most commonly used for sampling superficial sites such as the vagina and oropharynx. Moistening the swab tip by immersing in a fluid-enrichment medium may increase the sensitivity.

Rapid specimen transport to the laboratory is necessary to avoid desiccation. *C. albicans* can survive for at least 24 hours on a moist swab without loss of viability. It is better to use a transport medium for swabs whenever there may be a delay. Most well known transport media, such as Amies or Stuarts, are satisfactory for this purpose.

The most popular and useful agar culture media for primary isolation are versions of peptone-glucose or peptone-maltose agars, first described by Sabouraud in 1894. A concentration of live yeast cells of at least 10^3 per ml is necessary for reliable isolation on agar plates.

Identification of *Candida* species

Some differential isolation media, such as Nickerson's and Pagano–Levin's, contain indicator substances upon which *C. albicans* colonies differ in colour from other yeasts. Rapid identification of *C. albicans* is traditionally performed by the germ-tube test. *C. albicans* alone produces hyphal outgrowths when incubated at 37°C in serum for 2 hours. Assimilation and fermentation tests are used to differentiate other *Candida* species. A variety of commercial systems are available such as the API 20C kit. Antigenic and genotypic differentiation of isolates is also possible.

There is no reliable serological technique for diagnosing symptomatic VVC. A number of commercial companies have produced latex agglutination tests. These use polyclonal antibodies to detect soluble mannin antigens of multiple *Candida* strains. The tests may correlate more closely than cultures with symptomatic disease.

4.3 Differential diagnosis

The symptoms of vulval itch and vaginal discharge can be caused by a wide spectrum of other disorders including infective and non-infective genital disorders.

Causes of excessive vaginal discharge		
Vaginal infections	**Cervical infections**	**Other**
Candidosis	Chlamydia trachomatis	Physiological
Bacterial vaginosis	Gonorrhoea	Chemotrauma
Trichomoniasis	Genital herpes	Foreign body
		Fistulae
		Cervical polyp
		Malignancy

Bacterial vaginosis

This frequently recurring condition is more common than vaginal candidosis among STD clinic attenders and in some surveys of women presenting to family practitioners.

There is a disturbance in the normal bacterial flora of the vagina. Lactobacilli, the predominant flora, are replaced by a mixture of *Garnerella vaginalis* and anaerobic bacteria. Motile rod-shaped bacteria of the *Mobiluncus* species and high concentrations of genital mycoplasmas may also be present. Typically, the vaginal pH rises above 5.0.

Symptoms and signs

Although many women remain asymptomatic, others complain of an excessive, watery discharge with a pronounced fishy smell, which is often more apparent after sexual intercourse. There is usually little or no accompanying itch or dyspareunia. Urinary symptoms are usually absent although bacterial vaginosis may predispose to urinary-tract infection in women who have a high concentration of *Enterobacteria* as part of their abnormal vaginal flora.

Many laboratories do not routinely culture vaginal swabs for *G.vaginalis* and other bacterial species which are often fastidious in their culture requirements. In these circumstances, a vaginal swab which is reported as showing 'no pathogenic growth' may mislead the clinician.

Treatment of bacterial vaginosis		
Drug	**Regimen**	**Comments**
Metronidazole tablets	2 g p.o. single dose 400 mg bid p.o. for 5–7 days	Nausea and vomiting common Take after food
Metronidazole pessaries/ suppositories	1 g for 4 days Intravaginal insertion	Avoid alcohol during treatment Avoid in first trimester of pregnancy
Clindamycin 2% cream	Insert intravaginally for 7 days	
Ampicilllin	500 mg qid for 7 days	Use in first trimester of pregnancy

The majority of male partners have no signs or symptoms although some have a mild non-gonococcal urethritis or balanitis. In women with recurrent bacterial vaginosis, it is advisable to see the partner and offer epidemiological treatment with metronidazole. Because bacterial vaginosis often recurs soon after the resumption of sexual intercourse (possibly related to the stimulatory effect of semen on the causative organisms), the use of condoms throughout the next menstrual cycle to allow a full restoration of normal bacterial flora is recommended.

Trichomoniasis
This sexually transmitted condition is caused by the unicellular, motile, flagellated protozoan, *Trichomonas vaginalis*. It is more common in adolescents and perimenopausal women but has become less common in many developing countries during the past decade.

Symptoms and signs

Although asymptomatic trichomonal infection may persist for many years, the majority of infected women will develop a profuse, foul-smelling vaginal discharge, associated vulval soreness and swelling, and urinary symptoms of dysuria and frequency.

Typically, a pronounced diffuse vulvitis often accompanied by oedema and intertrigo are present together with pronounced vaginitis and petechial haemorrhages of the vaginal wall and ectocervix ('strawberry cervix').

Trichomoniasis frequently occurs with other sexually transmitted diseases, which should also be investigated. Both the patient and her partner should be treated. Metronidazole is the treatment of first choice in the UK.

Treatment failures are frequently due to reinfection. Resistance to metronidazole remains uncommon. If it does occur, the combination of systemic and topical metronidazole with a broad spectrum antibiotic is usually effective. Rarely, intravenous therapy has to be used.

Treatment of trichomoniasis		
Drug	**Regimen**	**Comments**
Metronidazole tablets	2 g p.o. single dose 400 mg bid p.o. for 5–7 days	Nausea and vomiting common Take after food
Metronidazole pessaries/ suppositories	1 g for 4 days Intravaginal insertion	Avoid alcohol during treatment Avoid in first trimester of pregnancy
Clotrimazole	100 mg for 7–14 days Intravaginal insertion	Useful for metronidazole-resistant cases Symptomatic relief in first trimester of pregnancy
Acetarsol pessaries/ suppositories	1 nightly for 14 days	Useful for metronidazole-resistant cases

Other infective causes of excessive vaginal discharge

Chlamydia trachomatis is the most common sexually transmitted pathogen in developed countries. In men, it is the cause of 30–60% of cases of non-gonococcal urethritis and the most common cause of epididymitis in younger men. In women, early infection is often asymptomatic although 'thrush-like' symptoms are often seen. Ascending infections cause pelvic inflammatory disease and may lead to infertility. Vertically transmitted infections cause neonatal ophthalmia and infant pneumonitis.

Clinical diagnosis is unreliable, although follicular cervicitis and hypertrophic cervical ectopy with marked contact bleeding is typical. Specific culture or antigen detection tests for *C. trachomatis* should be employed routinely in the investigation of young women presenting with genital symptoms.

Treatment is with either tetracycline or erythromycin for 7–14 days. Partners should also be treated.

Gonorrhoea has become less common in the UK during the past decade but it remains frequent in many developing countries. The clinical features and complications are similar to those of chlamydial infections. Antibiotic resistance is now common in many countries. Referral for specialist advice and management is advisable in countries where specialist services for the management of STDs exist.

The first episode of genital herpes, whether caused by herpes simplex virus type 1 or type 2, usually presents as vulval disease. Cervicitis, of variable severity, is also present and may result in an excessive discharge. It is unusual for this to occur without painful vulval and introital ulcers which cause more pronounced symptoms. *C. albicans* is a common superinfection of genital ulcers.

Vulval conditions

A wide variety of vulval infective and non-infective conditions may present in a similar fashion to, predispose to, or co-exist with VVC. These include infestations, for example scabies or pediculosis, and infections such as genital human papilloma virus infection, molluscum contagiosum, tinea cruris and intertrigo secondary to vaginitis or cervicitis.

Pruritus, soreness, vulval burning, and superficial dyspareunia may also be caused by a large number of dermatological conditions:

- contact dermatitis

- dermatitis medicamentosa

- lichen simplex

- intertrigo

- seborrhoeic eczema

- flexural psoriasis

- apocrine acne

- lichen planus

- lichen sclerosus

- pemphigus vulgaris

- Behçets syndrome

- erythema multiforme

- vulval Crohn's disease

- fixed drug eruption

These symptoms may occasionally have a psychosexual basis.

The diagnosis of vulval dermatoses is often difficult. The normal characteristics are modified by moistness, tissue laxity, scratching, superimposed infection, and topical medications. Examination of the entire skin, mucous membranes, the scalp, and nails may give clues to the diagnosis. Vulval biopsy may be necessary.

4.4 Genital candidosis in the male

Asymptomatic candidal colonization, especially in uncircumcised men, is more common than symptomatic disease.

Penile candidosis is nearly always associated with infection in the female partner. It can also be seen in immunocompetent gay men as a consequence of orogenital transmission of *C. albicans*. The majority of patients will complain of an itchy penile rash appearing shortly after intercourse. It usually resolves spontaneously in a few days. Examination reveals a punctate balanitis which is later associated with some desquamation of the glans and prepuce.

Insulin-dependent diabetic males may present with a phimosis and fissuring of the foreskin. Cheesy, mycotic plaques will be found on gentle retraction of the foreskin.

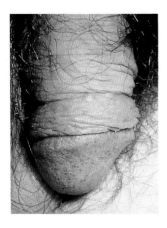

Candidosis in the male showing the presence of punctate balanitis

5 DRUG TREATMENT OF VVC

A wide variety of antifungal compounds are active against *Candida* species, most of which are suitable for topical application only.

Antifungal agents active against *Candida* species		
	Topical	**Oral**
Polyenes	Amphotericin B Candidacin Natamycin Nystatin	
Azole derivatives	Clotrimazole Miconazole Econazole Isoconazole Fenticonazole Butaconazole Tioconazole Terconazole	Ketoconazole
Triazoles		Fluconazole Itraconazole
Pyrimidines		Flucytosine

Topical agents fall into two major chemical classes: the polyenes and the azole derivatives.

5.1 Polyene antifungals
These are natural products of filamentous bacteria, usually *Streptomyces* species. Although over 100 polyenes are known, only four are routinely used in clinical practice: amphotericin B, nysatin, candidacin and natamycin.

Mode of action
Polyene drugs have a selective toxicity for fungal cell membranes, altering their permeability. They have a high avidity

for sterol binding, especially ergosterol. Cell-wall polysaccharides can act as barriers to penetration of polyenes.

Adverse effects
Side effects of treatment are uncommon although local irritation has been reported. The main patient complaint is the staining of underwear by pessary residue.

Amphotericin B
Amphotericin B when administered intravenously and intrathecally is mainly used for treatment of life-threatening systemic *Candida* infections, and rarely, if ever, in the treatment of VVC. It causes hypersensitivity reactions and has renal and hepatic toxicity. Topical applications for oral, genital and cutaneous candidosis are available in some countries.

Chemical structure of amphotericin B

Chemistry: $C_{47}H_{73}O_{17}$
Molecular weight = 924 Da

Nystatin
The drug was originally named after the New York State Antifungal Laboratory, where it was developed. It is the most widely used of the polyene antifungal agents used in the treatment of VVC and is available in the form of vaginal pessaries/suppositories, effervescent vaginal tablets, vaginal cream, and as topical cream or gel for application to the vulva. (The cream may damage latex condoms or diaphragms but the gel does not). It is also available as a suspension or pastilles for the treatment of oral candidosis, and as tablets

for the eradication of *Candida* species from the gut. The drug is not absorbed from the GI tract and has no systemic action. Treatment of acute vaginitis with nystatin usually gives rapid symptom relief although in order to achieve mycological cure rates of 70–80%, 7–14 days of treatment is required.

Candidacin

This is also too toxic for systemic use. It has been used to treat vaginal candidosis but less commonly than nystatin.

Natamycin

This topical agent is available as a 2% cream or 25 mg vaginal tablets for the treatment of vaginal candidosis. It appears to be less effective against *Candida* than other topical polyene species. Some activity against *Trichomonas vaginalis* has also been reported.

5.2 Azole antifungals

Azole antifungals		
First-generation	**Second-generation**	**Third-generation**
Clotrimazole	Ketoconazole	Fluconazole ⌒) (Diflaca)
Miconazole		Itraconazole
Econazole		
Isoconazole		

These include three generations of antifungal compound.

The first topical azole derivatives, clotrimazole and miconazole, appeared in 1969. Ketoconazole was introduced in 1979 as the first orally active azole antifungal. More recently, the triazoles, fluconazole and itraconazole, have been widely used for oral treatment of vaginal candidosis.

In the initial studies of topical imidazole antifungals, treatment courses of 5–7 days gave slight improvements in clinical and mycological efficacy compared with nystatin. Subsequent studies of the treatment of acute VVC have shown that almost identical cure rates of 80–90% can be produced with shorter treatment courses of 1–3 days.

Mode of action

All azole antifungals block the synthesis of ergosterol by inhibiting a 14-alpha demethylation step in fungal sterol biosynthesis mediated by the enzyme cytochrome P_{450}. This action is mainly fungistatic and particularly affects the ability of *C. albicans* to produce hyphal forms. They also exert fungicidal effects at high concentrations by directly damaging yeast membranes.

The development of *C. albicans* resistance to azoles is highly unusual but there are reports following protracted drug exposure. Resistant strains usually show cross-resistance to all other azole derivatives.

Topical azole drugs

There is little difference in efficacy between the topical azole drugs. Prescribing choice is mainly based upon physician familiarity, cost, and patient preference for different formulations. At 7 days post-treatment, over 90% of women will demonstrate clinical improvement and 80–95% mycological success. Symptomatic relapse occurs in 10–15% of women and recolonization by yeasts in 20–30% of individuals at 28 days post-treatment.

When vulval symptoms are marked, concomitant use of antifungal creams is often advised. There is no convincing evidence that this produces better short- or long-term cure rates but it may produce more rapid relief of itch and burning. The use of a steroid-containing antifungal cream may be preferred where there is marked vulval oedema or coexisting vulval eczema.

Adverse effects

Side effects of treatment are uncommon although all may cause local symptoms of irritation and burning, with signs erythema and oedema.

Ketoconazole

Ketonazole is supplied as 200 mg tablets or suspension, taken with food by mouth. Absorption is dependent upon gastric acidity. In acute VVC, the standard dosage is 200 mg

Topical azole antifungals		
Drug	**Formulation**	**Dosage**
Clotrimazole	100 mg vaginal tablet	1 tablet x 6 nights
	200 mg vaginal tablet	1 tablet x 3 nights
	500 mg vaginal tablet	1 tablet x 1 night
	Cream 1%	5 g x 7–14 nights
	Cream 10%	5 g x 1 night
Miconazole	100 mg vaginal pessary/suppository	1 pessary/suppository x 7 nights
	200 mg vaginal pessary/suppository	1 pessary/suppository x 3 nights
	Ovules 1.2 g in fatty base	1 ovule x 1 night
	Impregnated tampons	1 tampon x 5 nights
	Cream 2%	5 g x 7 nights
Econazole	150 mg vaginal pessary/suppository	1 pessary/suppository x 3 nights
Butaconazole	2% cream	5 g x 3 nights
Isoconazole	2% cream	2 pessaries/suppositories x 1 night
Fenticonazole	2% cream	5 g x 3 nights
Tioconazole	6.5% cream	5 g x 1 night
Terconazole	2% cream	5 g x 3 nights

twice daily for 5 days. A 2% topical cream is also available for topical anogenital use.

The main indications for use in *Candida* infections are onychomycosis and chronic mucocutaneous candidosis, but it is used as a prophylactic agent in immunocompromised patients.

In acute *Candida* vulvovaginosis, ketoconazole 200 mg twice daily for 5 days has at least equal efficacy to topical azole therapy. Concerns about hepatotoxicity have diminished clinician enthusiasm for long-term oral ketoconazole treatment.

Adverse effects

Unlike topical agents, the drug is contraindicated in pregnancy because teratogenic effects have been shown in animals. Ketoconazole is highly bound to plasma proteins. The drug inhibits some hepatic enzymes and serious interactions have been reported with cyclosporin, anticoagulants, terfenadine and a number of other drugs. Nausea and skin rashes also occur; gynaecomastia and inhibition of testosterone synthesis have been reported after prolonged therapy in men. Hepatotoxicity, sometimes fatal, is well recognized and occurs with a prevalence of 1 : 10 000. It is more common in women aged over 40, and occurs after 11–168 days of treatment with an average daily dosage of 200 mg. Transient abnormalities in liver function tests occur in approximately 10% of patients. The drug is contraindicated in those with known hepatic dysfunction.

Fluconazole

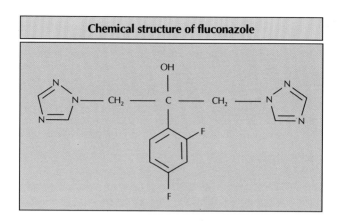

Chemical structure of fluconazole

Fluconazole is a bistriazole drug which is rapidly absorbed after oral administration, achieving peak plasma levels about 4 hours later. The oral bioavailability is over 90%; food does not significantly affect absorption. The mean plasma half-life is about 30 hours after a single 150 mg oral dose (in the figure shown below). The drug is largely excreted unchanged in the urine.

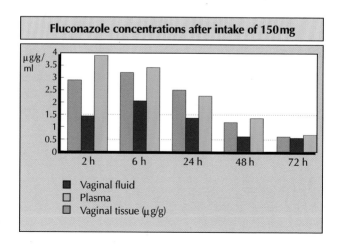

Fluconazole concentrations after intake of 150 mg

- Vaginal fluid
- Plasma
- Vaginal tissue (μg/g)

Fluconazole has low protein binding and is widely distributed. Vaginal tissue levels are similar to those in plasma. The levels achieved after a single 150 mg dosage remain in excess of the minimum inhibitory concentration of fluconazole to most strains of *C. albicans* for about 72 hours.

Adverse effects

Fluconazole has a high degree of selectivity for fungal cytochrome P_{450} enzymes and a negligible effect upon the corresponding human enzymes. Side effects are uncommon. Nausea, headache and abdominal discomfort are most often reported. Hypersensitivity rash can also occur. The drug can prolong prothrombin times in patients receiving warfarin and also prolongs the serum half-life of tolbutamide. No clinically significant interactions with oral contraceptive preparations are reported. The drug is not recommended for use in either pregnant women or lactating mothers.

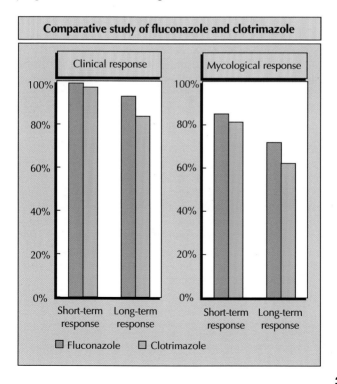

Comparative study of fluconazole and clotrimazole

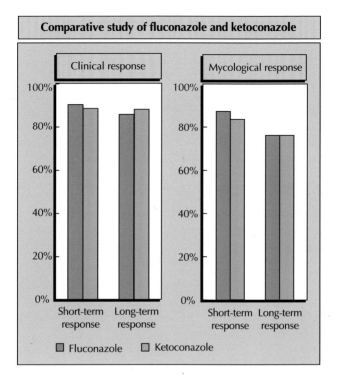

Comparative study of fluconazole and ketoconazole

A comparative trial of a single 150 mg oral dose of fluconazole with 3-day intravaginal treatment (using 200 mg clotrimazole pessaries/suppositories for the treatment of acute vaginal candidosis) showed more rapid onset and complete relief of symptoms with fluconazole (see figure opposite). Although short-term clinical and mycological cure rates were similar, long-term clinical and mycological response rates (assessed at 28 days after treatment) were better in the fluconazole-treated patients. There was a marked patient preference for oral treatment.

In another study in which single-dose 150 mg fluconazole was compared with 5-day treatment with oral ketoconazole 200 mg twice daily, the short-term and long-term clinical assessments were similar in both treatment groups (see figure above).

Itraconazole

Itraconazole is a large, complex azole molecule which has a high tissue affinity. It does not inhibit testicular or adrenal biosynthesis. It has a wide spectrum of antifungal activity and is useful in the treatment of superficial tinea infections in addition to systemic mycoses.

Drug absorption after oral dosage is improved when administered with a meal. Peak plasma concentrations are reached within 1.5–4 hours. It is widely distributed, achieving concentrations in some tissues 10-fold higher than plasma concentrations. It has a high affinity for sebum and keratinocytes. Itraconazole undergoes extensive hepatic metabolism and is excreted in the urine in an inactive form. The serum elimination half-life after a single oral dose of 100 mg is 20 hours but increases with dose and continuing administration after two weeks, to 34–42 hours.

In the treatment of acute vaginal candidosis, the total dose is more important than the duration of therapy. A minimum of 400 mg, given in two doses 12 hours apart, is required to maintain a mycological cure in 80% of patients one month after treatment.

Adverse effects

The drug is well tolerated by most patients. Gastrointestinal disturbances are the most common adverse effect and headache may also occur. The drug should be avoided in pregnancy. Caution is necessary if the drug is administered to patients with liver disease.

In a multicentre comparative study, in which patients were treated with either itraconazole 200 mg twice daily for one day or a single 500 mg clotrimazole tablet inserted intravaginally, the mycological cure rates 5–10 days after treatment were 74% in the itraconazole group and 72% in the clotrimazole group. Thirty to forty days after treatment, the overall mycological cure was 51% and 50%, respectively, for the two treatments, with 30% of the itraconazole group and 29% of the clotrimazole group demonstrating mycological relapse.

Flucytosine

This fluorinated pyrimidine drug was initially developed as a potential anticancer agent. It is phosphorylated within fungal cells to an active compound which interferes with DNA synthesis. It inhibits many yeasts *in vitro* but is much less inhibitory against filamentous strains such as *C. albicans*. The drug is most often used in the treatment of systemic mycoses, often in association with amphotericin B. It is sometimes used in resistant *C. glabrata* infections. Flucytosine is well absorbed from the gut and is available as an intraveneous infusion.

Adverse effects

Toxicity is uncommon although blood dyscrasias and hepatic toxicity have been reported. GI disturbances and skin rashes also occur.

The high prevalence of both primary and secondary resistance to flucytosine should restrict its use in treating superficial *Candida* infections.

Topical or oral treatment of acute vaginal candidosis?

The choice of oral or topical treatment in acute VVC is largely based upon individual patient and physician preference and cost. There may be marginal therapeutic advantages to oral therapy. Although topical agents are considerably cheaper than either fluconazole or itraconazole there is no need for concomitant topical antifungal treatment with these oral drugs.

5.3 Patient self-help

Vulval discomfort can be relieved by salt baths. Advice on the maintenance of genital hygiene, the establishment of correct toilet habit to prevent reinfection from the anorectum, and avoidance of any precipitating factors such as cosmetic or deodorant skin sensitizers may reduce the risk of clinical relapse. The use of vaginal lubricant gels may benefit women with dyspareunia. Steam ironing of underwear will kill yeasts which persist on underwear after warm water laundering. Concurrent treatment of the asymptomatic male partner is not normally required. Provision of an information leaflet to patients is often as useful reminder of the physician's advice. This can give further details of self-help measures (see Appendix).

5.4 Treatment failure

Under laboratory conditions, it is possible to induce resistance to antifungal drugs in many different isolates of *Candida*. Resistance is, however, very uncommon in clinical isolates from immunocompetent hosts and is more often of clinical significance in isolates from immunocompromised patients, especially those with granulocytopenia. True resistance to antifungal treatment is rare with *C. albicans* in otherwise healthy patients. In persistent infections, a longer topical treatment course or use of oral treatment will usually be successful. Antifungal sensitivity tests can give some guidance to the selection of further treatment of difficult cases.

Non-*albicans* strains of yeasts are more likely to fail to respond to azole therapy. *C. glabrata* and *S. cerevisiae* infections require special consideration.

Azole-resistant *Candida* glabrata

C. glabrata causes around 5% of VVC cases. It does not form germ-tubes, which results in the absence of filamentous elements on microscopy. Although these infections are often mild, the organism may rapidly develop resistance to topical azole drugs and oral triazoles, resulting in persistent vaginitis. In these cases, successful treatment with nystatin pessaries/ suppositories nightly for 14 days, boric acid gelatin capsules, and 1% gentian violet has been reported. Nevertheless, no single treatment is always effective and these cases can constitute a major challenge to the clinician.

Saccharomyces cerevisiae vaginitis

This is a rare condition causing less than 1% of yeast vaginitis. *S. cerevisiae* is used extensively in the brewing and baking industries. Colonization of the respiratory and urinary tracts and systemic infections with *Saccharomyces* species have been reported in immunocompromised patients.

Clinical infection with *S. cerevisiae* is indistinguishable from that caused by other yeasts. It most often occurs as part of a chronic syndrome in patients with local and systemic predisposing conditions. Microscopy of vaginal secretions reveals blastospores in the absence of filamentous elements. Response to short courses of topical azole drugs or oral fluconazole is poor. Treatment may need to be prolonged. Suggested regimens include clotrimazole 100 mg vaginal tablet for 7–10 days, boric acid 600 mg capsules for 7–10 days, oral keto-conazole 400 mg daily for 14 days. Successful treatment with nystatin pessaries/ suppositories for 14 days has also been reported.

Chronic or recurrent VVC

Persistent or recurrent genital symptoms are caused by *C. albicans* and other yeasts in up to 10% of affected women. It is essential to confirm the diagnosis by both clinical assessment and laboratory investigation. Many women with self-declared or physician-diagnosed chronic candidosis based on history alone have been incorrectly diagnosed.

In those with confirmed persistent or recurrent candidosis, assessment should be made of correctable predisposing factors. It is unusual to find a significant underlying pathology in otherwise healthy patients. Laboratory investigations should be minimized. Routine haematological and biochemical screening and urinalysis is justifiable. Glucose tolerance tests rarely reveal latent diabetes mellitus in patients without glycosuria unless there is a strong family history. Sources of vaginal reinfection with yeasts include

- external genitalia and skin
- clothing and other fomites
- Gastrointestinal tract
- male partner
- deeper layers of vagina

Significantly more women with recurring vaginitis within one month of oral fluconazole treatment have persistent rectal yeast colonization detected at short-term follow-up than those who remain infection-free. Nevertheless, previous studies have shown that the use of oral nystatin treatment to eradicate yeasts from the GI tract fails to prevent recurrence.

Simultaneous rectal colonization with identical yeast species occurs in 75% of affected women. Similarly, 65% of recurrences within 3 months of treatment are from an identical yeast strain. Clinical relapse correlates with the failure to eradicate rectal colonization after a single dose of oral antifungal treatment.

However, symptoms recur in the absence of rectal colonization in 50% of affected women.

Male partners

About two-thirds of the male partners of affected women can be found to have the same biotype of yeast residing on the penis or the mouth. Peno-vaginal or oro-genital sexual contact may be a source of reinfection in about 10% of affected women. Studies have shown that partners of infected women have a fourfold higher penile colonization rate than controls. In most cases neither topical nor systemic antifungal treatment of male partners influences recurrence rates in affected women.

Fomites

C. albicans can survive on moist surfaces, in oil-water based cosmetics, and on diaphragms and toothbrushes. The yeast on contaminated underwear is not killed by low temperature washing. The use of prewash soaks in candidacidal solutions or steam ironing of underwear can help eradicate reinfection from this source.

Vaginal relapse

Vaginal yeasts can penetrate through to the deeper layers of vaginal epithelium, where they are relatively impervious to topical antifungal agents. Low concentrations of residual yeasts ($< 10^3$/ml) may fail to grow on conventional cultures in the immediate post-treatment period. Yeasts from the deeper layers may subsequently emerge to recolonize the vaginal lumen.

Attention to all of these potential sources is important in managing individual patients.

Management of recurrent VVC

Patients can now be reassured that it is possible in virtually every case to eradicate yeasts from the genital tract and control the symptoms of recurrent VVC. This is achieved by an initial sustained course of antifungal therapy, followed by intermittent prophylactic therapy.

There are a number of different regimens, the choice of which must be tailored to the needs of the individual. Initial regimens include either clotrimazole 100 mg or miconazole 100 mg pessaries/suppositories for 6–12 nights. Many clinicians prefer oral anti-fungal therapy — suitable initiating regimens used in acute episodes include 150 mg fluconazole given as a single dose, or itraconazole 200 mg daily for 3 days. In some women it may be necessary to repeat these oral treatments at intervals of 4 to 7 days.

Suppressive antifungals may then be administered once a week and gradually reduced to fortnightly (day 7 and day 21 of the cycle) and monthly intervals (day 21 is preferable, especially in women with premenstrual symptom exacerbation). The standard dose of itraconazole is 200 mg taken twice for one day with 12 hours separation between doses. Examples of suppressive single-dose therapy include clotrimazole 500 mg vaginal tablet, econazole 150 mg pessary/suppository or fluconazole 150 mg orally.

After the symptoms have been completely suppressed for 3–6 months, therapy can be withdrawn to allow reassessment. In at least half of the treated patients the previous symptom pattern will not resume. Suppressive treatment can be recommenced in women who do undergo relapse.

5.5 Alternative treatments

Gentian violet

This was a mainstay of treatment before the development of antifungal drugs. Crystal violet paint 0.5% is licensed for use only on unbroken skin and is no longer recommended for application on mucosal surfaces.

Lactobacillus

Vaginal lactobacilli offer a degree of non-specific protection against infection by producing an acid environment that inhibits the growth of many bacterial pathogens. Lactobacilli inhibit the growth of *C. albicans*. It has also been suggested that some women obtain some benefit from exogenous lactobacilli, in the form of either oral preparations containing lactobacilli or, more usually, dairy products such as plain live yoghurt applied to the vulva or inserted into the vagina.

There is little scientific evidence for the efficacy of these approaches; the vaginal pH is not elevated in most women suffering from candidosis and lactobacilli are usually abundant in Gram-stained smears.

It is more likely, but not proven, that exogenous lactobacilli might be of some benefit in women suffering from bacterial vaginosis, although many women testify to the soothing effect of cold yoghurt applied to the inflamed genitals in acute candidosis.

Garlic

Allicin, which is also responsible for the odour of garlic, has antimicrobial action against *Candida* species and various bacterial species. It has been used in a variety of traditional herbal preparations. There is no convincing evidence of therapeutic effect. Garlic cloves should never be applied directly to the vagina or vulva because they are intense mucosal irritants and can cause severe ulceration.

Other topical preparations

A wide variety of other topical agents, including hydrogaphen, potassium sorbate, povidone iodine and proprionic acid, have been used in VVC. There is no scientific evidence that they have advantages over specific antifungal therapies.

Immunotherapy

The recognition that there may be specific defects in the cellular immune response to *Candida* antigens in some women with recurrent VVC has led some investigators to attempt immunotherapy as an alternative to suppressive anti-fungal intervention.

Hyposensitization with a commercially available *C. albicans* antigen in an uncontrolled trial has been reported to give encouraging results.

Further Reading

1. Soll DR. Molecular and cell biology of *Candida* pathogenesis. In *Molecular And Cell Biology Of Sexually Transmitted Disease* edited by Wright D and Ackland L. London: Chapman and Hall, 1992.

This book chapter provides an up-to-date account of knowledge concerning the biology, pathogenesis and epidemiology of *Candida* infections.

2. Odds FC. Candida *and Candidosis. A Review And Bibliography*. London: Bailliere Tindall, 1988.

This book gives a comprehensive review with a microbiological emphasis on all aspects of human *Candida* infections.

3. Sobel JD. Vulvovaginal Candidiasis. In *Sexually Transmitted Diseases 2nd edn* edited by Holmes KK, Mardh P-A, Sparling PF, *et al*. New York: McGraw Hill, 1990.

This is an excellent review of the subject by the foremost clinical researcher into genital candidosis in North America.

'Thrush' — A self-help guide
Advice leaflets for your patients

'Thrush' — A self-help guide

Vaginal candidosis (or vaginal candidiasis) is also known as thrush in many countries. It is extremely common and affects most women at some times in their lives. The condition is caused by a yeast, usually *Candida albicans*. This germ lives normally in the mouths or bowel of many people who are unaware of it, as it generally causes no harm. Sometimes, however, the yeast multiplies and causes symptoms such as mouth soreness or napkin rash. In women, the disease can affect the vulva and vagina and result in itching and soreness, which is often worse at night. Men may also develop symptoms after sex, which can give rise to an itchy rash appearing on the head of the penis.

How is vaginal thrush treated?

If you get an itch or a discharge which you have never had before, you should seek medical help. Salt baths will help reduce the discomfort until you see the doctor. The doctor will need to ask some questions about your symptoms and an examination is usually necessary. Tests of the vaginal secretions may be taken and sent to the laboratory.

Thrush is most often treated with local pessaries or suppositories. These are special tablets which are placed into the vagina (usually at night), where they will dissolve. To prevent daytime leakage and soiling of your underwear, it is wise to wear a minipad during the period of treatment. You may also be given some cream to apply to the outside skin. This will help to stop the itching. Some doctors use tablets taken by mouth to treat this infection. If this type of treatment is used, pessaries and creams are usually not necessary.

It is very important to complete the course of treatment. The symptoms often clear up *before the infection has completely gone*. If you stop treatment too soon, another outbreak is more likely.

How can thrush be prevented?

There is no simple solution to this question. The doctor may prescribe regular treatment to prevent further episodes in women who have very frequent attacks. But there are a number of things which you can do to help.

- Avoid tights, pantyhose, nylon underwear, tight leggings or jeans, and cycling pants. Wear skirts, cotton underwear, stockings or socks. These will help to prevent the genital area from becoming too warm and moist.

- Use pads rather than tampons when you have a menstrual period.

- Avoid perfumed soaps, vaginal deodorants, bubble bath and any other irritants such as disinfectants. The only additive you may use in the bath is simple salt. The amount which can be held in the palm of one hand is sufficient.

- Always wash and wipe from front to back after using the lavatory. This will help to prevent contamination of the genital area by yeasts or other germs which live in the bowel and around the anus.

- Use vaginal lubricants, e.g. KY jelly, during intercourse. Vaginal dryness is commonly caused by thrush and may persist after treatment. The friction of sexual intercourse may then cause minor damage to the vagina, which allows yeasts to cause further infection. The lubricant should be applied liberally to the vaginal entrance. Your partner may also apply this to the head of his penis.

- Some condoms contain a spermicide lubricant which can cause irritation. Some women will benefit from a change to 'hypoallergenic' condoms.

- It is advisable for your partner to be treated if you have had repeated attacks. His treatment will normally consist of the application of a cream to the penis for up to 7 days.

- There is little medical evidence that diet plays a part in allowing thrush to develop but a well-balanced diet is advised for all people. You should avoid too many sugary or starchy foods. If you are overweight, a sensible weight-reducing diet may help. Some women have found that applying plain live yoghurt onto the vulva or into the vaginal is soothing.

- Yeasts can survive the warm-wash cycle. They die rapidly when exposed to temperatures exceeding 50°C. To prevent reinfection from underwear, steam ironing is recommended.

Ask your doctor if either you or your partner have any further questions about the treatment or prevention of thrush

'Thrush' — A self-help guide

Vaginal candidosis (or vaginal candidiasis) is also known as thrush in many countries. It is extremely common and affects most women at some times in their lives. The condition is caused by a yeast, usually *Candida albicans*. This germ lives normally in the mouths or bowel of many people who are unaware of it, as it generally causes no harm. Sometimes, however, the yeast multiplies and causes symptoms such as mouth soreness or napkin rash. In women, the disease can affect the vulva and vagina and result in itching and soreness, which is often worse at night. Men may also develop symptoms after sex, which can give rise to an itchy rash appearing on the head of the penis.

How is vaginal thrush treated?

If you get an itch or a discharge which you have never had before, you should seek medical help. Salt baths will help reduce the discomfort until you see the doctor. The doctor will need to ask some questions about your symptoms and an examination is usually necessary. Tests of the vaginal secretions may be taken and sent to the laboratory.

Thrush is most often treated with local pessaries or suppositories. These are special tablets which are placed into the vagina (usually at night), where they will dissolve. To prevent daytime leakage and soiling of your underwear, it is wise to wear a minipad during the period of treatment. You may also be given some cream to apply to the outside skin. This will help to stop the itching. Some doctors use tablets taken by mouth to treat this infection. If this type of treatment is used, pessaries and creams are usually not necessary.

It is very important to complete the course of treatment. The symptoms often clear up *before the infection has completely gone*. If you stop treatment too soon, another outbreak is more likely.

How can thrush be prevented?

There is no simple solution to this question. The doctor may prescribe regular treatment to prevent further episodes in women who have very frequent attacks. But there are a number of things which you can do to help.

- Avoid tights, pantyhose, nylon underwear, tight leggings or jeans, and cycling pants. Wear skirts, cotton underwear, stockings or socks. These will help to prevent the genital area from becoming too warm and moist.

- Use pads rather than tampons when you have a menstrual period.

- Avoid perfumed soaps, vaginal deodorants, bubble bath and any other irritants such as disinfectants. The only additive you may use in the bath is simple salt. The amount which can be held in the palm of one hand is sufficient.

- Always wash and wipe from front to back after using the lavatory. This will help to prevent contamination of the genital area by yeasts or other germs which live in the bowel and around the anus.

- Use vaginal lubricants, e.g. KY jelly, during intercourse. Vaginal dryness is commonly caused by thrush and may persist after treatment. The friction of sexual intercourse may then cause minor damage to the vagina, which allows yeasts to cause further infection. The lubricant should be applied liberally to the vaginal entrance. Your partner may also apply this to the head of his penis.

- Some condoms contain a spermicide lubricant which can cause irritation. Some women will benefit from a change to 'hypoallergenic' condoms.

- It is advisable for your partner to be treated if you have had repeated attacks. His treatment will normally consist of the application of a cream to the penis for up to 7 days.

- There is little medical evidence that diet plays a part in allowing thrush to develop but a well-balanced diet is advised for all people. You should avoid too many sugary or starchy foods. If you are overweight, a sensible weight-reducing diet may help. Some women have found that applying plain live yoghurt onto the vulva or into the vaginal is soothing.

- Yeasts can survive the warm-wash cycle. They die rapidly when exposed to temperatures exceeding 50°C. To prevent reinfection from underwear, steam ironing is recommended.

Ask your doctor if either you or your partner have any further questions about the treatment or prevention of thrush

'Thrush' — A self-help guide

Vaginal candidosis (or vaginal candidiasis) is also known as thrush in many countries. It is extremely common and affects most women at some times in their lives. The condition is caused by a yeast, usually *Candida albicans*. This germ lives normally in the mouths or bowel of many people who are unaware of it, as it generally causes no harm. Sometimes, however, the yeast multiplies and causes symptoms such as mouth soreness or napkin rash. In women, the disease can affect the vulva and vagina and result in itching and soreness, which is often worse at night. Men may also develop symptoms after sex, which can give rise to an itchy rash appearing on the head of the penis.

How is vaginal thrush treated?

If you get an itch or a discharge which you have never had before, you should seek medical help. Salt baths will help reduce the discomfort until you see the doctor. The doctor will need to ask some questions about your symptoms and an examination is usually necessary. Tests of the vaginal secretions may be taken and sent to the laboratory.

Thrush is most often treated with local pessaries or suppositories. These are special tablets which are placed into the vagina (usually at night), where they will dissolve. To prevent daytime leakage and soiling of your underwear, it is wise to wear a minipad during the period of treatment. You may also be given some cream to apply to the outside skin. This will help to stop the itching. Some doctors use tablets taken by mouth to treat this infection. If this type of treatment is used, pessaries and creams are usually not necessary.

It is very important to complete the course of treatment. The symptoms often clear up *before the infection has completely gone*. If you stop treatment too soon, another outbreak is more likely.

How can thrush be prevented?

There is no simple solution to this question. The doctor may prescribe regular treatment to prevent further episodes in women who have very frequent attacks. But there are a number of things which you can do to help.

- Avoid tights, pantyhose, nylon underwear, tight leggings or jeans, and cycling pants. Wear skirts, cotton underwear, stockings or socks. These will help to prevent the genital area from becoming too warm and moist.

- Use pads rather than tampons when you have a menstrual period.

- Avoid perfumed soaps, vaginal deodorants, bubble bath and any other irritants such as disinfectants. The only additive you may use in the bath is simple salt. The amount which can be held in the palm of one hand is sufficient.

- Always wash and wipe from front to back after using the lavatory. This will help to prevent contamination of the genital area by yeasts or other germs which live in the bowel and around the anus.

- Use vaginal lubricants, e.g. KY jelly, during intercourse. Vaginal dryness is commonly caused by thrush and may persist after treatment. The friction of sexual intercourse may then cause minor damage to the vagina, which allows yeasts to cause further infection. The lubricant should be applied liberally to the vaginal entrance. Your partner may also apply this to the head of his penis.

- Some condoms contain a spermicide lubricant which can cause irritation. Some women will benefit from a change to 'hypoallergenic' condoms.

- It is advisable for your partner to be treated if you have had repeated attacks. His treatment will normally consist of the application of a cream to the penis for up to 7 days.

- There is little medical evidence that diet plays a part in allowing thrush to develop but a well-balanced diet is advised for all people. You should avoid too many sugary or starchy foods. If you are overweight, a sensible weight-reducing diet may help. Some women have found that applying plain live yoghurt onto the vulva or into the vaginal is soothing.

- Yeasts can survive the warm-wash cycle. They die rapidly when exposed to temperatures exceeding 50°C. To prevent reinfection from underwear, steam ironing is recommended.

Ask your doctor if either you or your partner have any further questions about the treatment or prevention of thrush

'Thrush' — A self-help guide

Vaginal candidosis (or vaginal candidiasis) is also known as thrush in many countries. It is extremely common and affects most women at some times in their lives. The condition is caused by a yeast, usually *Candida albicans*. This germ lives normally in the mouths or bowel of many people who are unaware of it, as it generally causes no harm. Sometimes, however, the yeast multiplies and causes symptoms such as mouth soreness or napkin rash. In women, the disease can affect the vulva and vagina and result in itching and soreness, which is often worse at night. Men may also develop symptoms after sex, which can give rise to an itchy rash appearing on the head of the penis.

How is vaginal thrush treated?

If you get an itch or a discharge which you have never had before, you should seek medical help. Salt baths will help reduce the discomfort until you see the doctor. The doctor will need to ask some questions about your symptoms and an examination is usually necessary. Tests of the vaginal secretions may be taken and sent to the laboratory.

Thrush is most often treated with local pessaries or suppositories. These are special tablets which are placed into the vagina (usually at night), where they will dissolve. To prevent daytime leakage and soiling of your underwear, it is wise to wear a minipad during the period of treatment. You may also be given some cream to apply to the outside skin. This will help to stop the itching. Some doctors use tablets taken by mouth to treat this infection. If this type of treatment is used, pessaries and creams are usually not necessary.

It is very important to complete the course of treatment. The symptoms often clear up *before the infection has completely gone.* If you stop treatment too soon, another outbreak is more likely.

How can thrush be prevented?

There is no simple solution to this question. The doctor may prescribe regular treatment to prevent further episodes in women who have very frequent attacks. But there are a number of things which you can do to help.

- Avoid tights, pantyhose, nylon underwear, tight leggings or jeans, and cycling pants. Wear skirts, cotton underwear, stockings or socks. These will help to prevent the genital area from becoming too warm and moist.

- Use pads rather than tampons when you have a menstrual period.

- Avoid perfumed soaps, vaginal deodorants, bubble bath and any other irritants such as disinfectants. The only additive you may use in the bath is simple salt. The amount which can be held in the palm of one hand is sufficient.

- Always wash and wipe from front to back after using the lavatory. This will help to prevent contamination of the genital area by yeasts or other germs which live in the bowel and around the anus.

- Use vaginal lubricants, e.g. KY jelly, during intercourse. Vaginal dryness is commonly caused by thrush and may persist after treatment. The friction of sexual intercourse may then cause minor damage to the vagina, which allows yeasts to cause further infection. The lubricant should be applied liberally to the vaginal entrance. Your partner may also apply this to the head of his penis.

- Some condoms contain a spermicide lubricant which can cause irritation. Some women will benefit from a change to 'hypoallergenic' condoms.

- It is advisable for your partner to be treated if you have had repeated attacks. His treatment will normally consist of the application of a cream to the penis for up to 7 days.

- There is little medical evidence that diet plays a part in allowing thrush to develop but a well-balanced diet is advised for all people. You should avoid too many sugary or starchy foods. If you are overweight, a sensible weight-reducing diet may help. Some women have found that applying plain live yoghurt onto the vulva or into the vaginal is soothing.

- Yeasts can survive the warm-wash cycle. They die rapidly when exposed to temperatures exceeding $50^{o}C$. To prevent reinfection from underwear, steam ironing is recommended.

Ask your doctor if either you or your partner have any further questions about the treatment or prevention of thrush

'Thrush' — A self-help guide

Vaginal candidosis (or vaginal candidiasis) is also known as thrush in many countries. It is extremely common and affects most women at some times in their lives. The condition is caused by a yeast, usually *Candida albicans*. This germ lives normally in the mouths or bowel of many people who are unaware of it, as it generally causes no harm. Sometimes, however, the yeast multiplies and causes symptoms such as mouth soreness or napkin rash. In women, the disease can affect the vulva and vagina and result in itching and soreness, which is often worse at night. Men may also develop symptoms after sex, which can give rise to an itchy rash appearing on the head of the penis.

How is vaginal thrush treated?

If you get an itch or a discharge which you have never had before, you should seek medical help. Salt baths will help reduce the discomfort until you see the doctor. The doctor will need to ask some questions about your symptoms and an examination is usually necessary. Tests of the vaginal secretions may be taken and sent to the laboratory.

Thrush is most often treated with local pessaries or suppositories. These are special tablets which are placed into the vagina (usually at night), where they will dissolve. To prevent daytime leakage and soiling of your underwear, it is wise to wear a minipad during the period of treatment. You may also be given some cream to apply to the outside skin. This will help to stop the itching. Some doctors use tablets taken by mouth to treat this infection. If this type of treatment is used, pessaries and creams are usually not necessary.

It is very important to complete the course of treatment. The symptoms often clear up *before the infection has completely gone*. If you stop treatment too soon, another outbreak is more likely.

How can thrush be prevented?

There is no simple solution to this question. The doctor may prescribe regular treatment to prevent further episodes in women who have very frequent attacks. But there are a number of things which you can do to help.

- Avoid tights, pantyhose, nylon underwear, tight leggings or jeans, and cycling pants. Wear skirts, cotton underwear, stockings or socks. These will help to prevent the genital area from becoming too warm and moist.

- Use pads rather than tampons when you have a menstrual period.

- Avoid perfumed soaps, vaginal deodorants, bubble bath and any other irritants such as disinfectants. The only additive you may use in the bath is simple salt. The amount which can be held in the palm of one hand is sufficient.

- Always wash and wipe from front to back after using the lavatory. This will help to prevent contamination of the genital area by yeasts or other germs which live in the bowel and around the anus.

- Use vaginal lubricants, e.g. KY jelly, during intercourse. Vaginal dryness is commonly caused by thrush and may persist after treatment. The friction of sexual intercourse may then cause minor damage to the vagina, which allows yeasts to cause further infection. The lubricant should be applied liberally to the vaginal entrance. Your partner may also apply this to the head of his penis.

- Some condoms contain a spermicide lubricant which can cause irritation. Some women will benefit from a change to 'hypoallergenic' condoms.

- It is advisable for your partner to be treated if you have had repeated attacks. His treatment will normally consist of the application of a cream to the penis for up to 7 days.

- There is little medical evidence that diet plays a part in allowing thrush to develop but a well-balanced diet is advised for all people. You should avoid too many sugary or starchy foods. If you are overweight, a sensible weight-reducing diet may help. Some women have found that applying plain live yoghurt onto the vulva or into the vaginal is soothing.

- Yeasts can survive the warm-wash cycle. They die rapidly when exposed to temperatures exceeding 50°C. To prevent reinfection from underwear, steam ironing is recommended.

Ask your doctor if either you or your partner have any further questions about the treatment or prevention of thrush

'Thrush' — A self-help guide

Vaginal candidosis (or vaginal candidiasis) is also known as thrush in many countries. It is extremely common and affects most women at some times in their lives. The condition is caused by a yeast, usually *Candida albicans*. This germ lives normally in the mouths or bowel of many people who are unaware of it, as it generally causes no harm. Sometimes, however, the yeast multiplies and causes symptoms such as mouth soreness or napkin rash. In women, the disease can affect the vulva and vagina and result in itching and soreness, which is often worse at night. Men may also develop symptoms after sex, which can give rise to an itchy rash appearing on the head of the penis.

How is vaginal thrush treated?

If you get an itch or a discharge which you have never had before, you should seek medical help. Salt baths will help reduce the discomfort until you see the doctor. The doctor will need to ask some questions about your symptoms and an examination is usually necessary. Tests of the vaginal secretions may be taken and sent to the laboratory.

Thrush is most often treated with local pessaries or suppositories. These are special tablets which are placed into the vagina (usually at night), where they will dissolve. To prevent daytime leakage and soiling of your underwear, it is wise to wear a minipad during the period of treatment. You may also be given some cream to apply to the outside skin. This will help to stop the itching. Some doctors use tablets taken by mouth to treat this infection. If this type of treatment is used, pessaries and creams are usually not necessary.

It is very important to complete the course of treatment. The symptoms often clear up *before the infection has completely gone*. If you stop treatment too soon, another outbreak is more likely.

How can thrush be prevented?

There is no simple solution to this question. The doctor may prescribe regular treatment to prevent further episodes in women who have very frequent attacks. But there are a number of things which you can do to help.

- Avoid tights, pantyhose, nylon underwear, tight leggings or jeans, and cycling pants. Wear skirts, cotton underwear, stockings or socks. These will help to prevent the genital area from becoming too warm and moist.

- Use pads rather than tampons when you have a menstrual period.

- Avoid perfumed soaps, vaginal deodorants, bubble bath and any other irritants such as disinfectants. The only additive you may use in the bath is simple salt. The amount which can be held in the palm of one hand is sufficient.

- Always wash and wipe from front to back after using the lavatory. This will help to prevent contamination of the genital area by yeasts or other germs which live in the bowel and around the anus.

- Use vaginal lubricants, e.g. KY jelly, during intercourse. Vaginal dryness is commonly caused by thrush and may persist after treatment. The friction of sexual intercourse may then cause minor damage to the vagina, which allows yeasts to cause further infection. The lubricant should be applied liberally to the vaginal entrance. Your partner may also apply this to the head of his penis.

- Some condoms contain a spermicide lubricant which can cause irritation. Some women will benefit from a change to 'hypoallergenic' condoms.

- It is advisable for your partner to be treated if you have had repeated attacks. His treatment will normally consist of the application of a cream to the penis for up to 7 days.

- There is little medical evidence that diet plays a part in allowing thrush to develop but a well-balanced diet is advised for all people. You should avoid too many sugary or starchy foods. If you are overweight, a sensible weight-reducing diet may help. Some women have found that applying plain live yoghurt onto the vulva or into the vaginal is soothing.

- Yeasts can survive the warm-wash cycle. They die rapidly when exposed to temperatures exceeding 50°C. To prevent reinfection from underwear, steam ironing is recommended.

Ask your doctor if either you or your partner have any further questions about the treatment or prevention of thrush